This book is merely a mosaic of ideas and concepts that have been passed on to me by amazing mentors and peers. I would like to formally express my deepest gratitude to them and their teachers before them... "We stand on each other's shoulders."

Especially Scott Sonnon, Gwint Fisher, Alaina Sawaya, and the entire Rmax/TacFit Legion.

Jason Hawkins, Jared Jessup, Derik Perry, Eli Knight, Clay Mayfield and the entire Gracie Jiu Jitsu Family.

Nicole Brown and the Iyengar Yoga Community.

Summer Huntington and Flow State of Mind Coaching.

Thank you to my parents Bret and Linda Beegle for believing in me, not letting me drown in my own stupidity, and giving me more second chances than I deserve.

To my other parents Tom and Laura Merz. Your continued and generous support has allowed our family to plant strong roots and grow into something better than I ever imagined. Thanks for putting up with me.

To the Seva Tribe. You motivate me more than you will ever know. This is all because of your support. Thanks for being the best guinea pigs. You will never have a fan bigger than me.

And a huge thanks to my editor Suzanne Clinton.
You're my "Ace in the hole"!

Check out her services at
www.clintoncreative.com

Live Better Die Slower Book Series

Copyright © 2019 by Eric Romanak

Seva Fitness

ISBN: 9781094674643

To:

E+D=M2

This equation saved my life. You are my world.

5

FOREWORD

"Don't take life too seriously. You will never get out alive."

- Elbert Hubbard

Since I got into the health and fitness business I have always been seen as a bit unconventional. I was a terrible athlete as a kid, and had the genetics of a wet towel. I am tall, lanky, have the body of a distance runner, and should've gotten braces when I was a kid. In short, I have never had the classic look of a chiseled, square-jawed personal trainer, nor have I ever coached people like a typical trainer either.

For decades I walked around in a muffin top - man boob fat jacket, and when I first started to teach fitness classes I was still hanging onto a bit of "my old self" around the waistline. At one point, there was a middle-aged lady who came to my first class. She kept coming back for a few weeks. As a new instructor, anyone who came to your class more than once gave you a much-needed confidence boost. One day she tried to give me a compliment in front of the class by saying, "The thing I like about you Eric is you don't look like a personal trainer, you're just a normal looking guy." She said this as she gave me a Vanna White arm wave directed at my torso. Cue the trombone slide… I was mortified. Inside, I was still battling with the image of the fat kid I used to be growing up, and that kid still had a space in my head. Truth be told, he still does. It's just a much smaller space he rents now. But she was right. I was just a normal guy, and that's who I've been preaching fitness is for: normal people.

As we start, it's really important that we are clear about one thing. I'm just a regular guy, a guy who is trying to figure shit out like the rest of us, and that's all I will ever be. While I love growing, reaching new goals and doing things I've never been able to do before, I will never be anything other than a person walking his own path. Just like all my clients. Just like you.

As a health coach I often get lumped into a certain stereotype, one that assumes I live some kind of near perfect hyper-disciplined life, and that I look down on people when they eat unhealthy foods or miss a workout. Let me just say this right off the bat: screw sainthood. I think Billy Joel said it best in Only the Good Die Young, "I'd rather laugh with the sinners than cry with the saints. The sinners are much more fun." Despite my deep core belief that health is a critical foundation to have in your life, and injecting functional discomfort in our lives is a big key to happiness, it still has to be put in a realistic context.

Living an overly restrictive life is not the same as living a healthy life.

There was a time in my life when I thought the intense discipline and purity of living life like a monk was somehow going to solve all my problems, but it didn't make me happy. It made me feel more in control (which was a delusion), but it pushed me farther away from people I cared about and made me a neurotic mess. In the end it was just another version of me trying to escape from my pain. It was just another addiction.

I'm not the kind of guy that advocates health as some kind of quest for purity.

Don't get me wrong, discipline is a huge part of my life, but I had to grow into it. In addition, I still like to have pancakes and lattes every once in a while. I am on my own journey, just like you, and I still have plenty of my own baggage to still unpack. I merely teach tools that were taught to me, and it's up to you to apply them as you see fit. They are simple things that made a big difference for me as well as for the people who gave them to me. Ultimately, they were designed to make us feel a little bit better as we walk the earth in our own unique skin suit.

My claim to try and help others is straightforward; I was in a lot of pain at one time in my life, because I refused to face it. I always tried to take the easiest path, and because of it I was falling behind. I was so incredibly lucky to have some amazing people cross my path. They had a very unique perspective that I needed to hear, and even more importantly to see it in action. It helped me start to move my needle, and now I have a strong internal need to pay it forward. But most importantly, I try, to the best of my ability, to live the things I believe in. I'm not perfect, and I have often been blinded by my ego, but I work hard as hell and course correct when I realize I need to. Otherwise I can't sleep at night.

I don't think I've done anything remarkable in my life other than I keep picking myself back up and moving forward.

These are crazy times, and there's some ugly stuff happening in the world. On an elemental level the world needs some more light to fight back some of the darkness these days. The amazing teachers and mentors in my life understood they were bearers of a torch which carried a kind of eternal flame. They graciously and selflessly lit my torch, and I hope to maybe light yours in some small way. Then it will be your turn. That's the way light overcomes the dark… it just stays lit.

The bullseye I'm aiming for in this life is to be able to say on my deathbed,

"I played the hand I was dealt the best I knew how, lived the life I earned, and tried to leave the world a little better."

Now I'm looking to help people who want that too.

I will be up front and save you time by telling you this, no book, diet or fitness program is going to penetrate your life or behavior cycle unless you are ready for it. By that, I don't mean you finally have time in your schedule to start a fitness program. That very rarely will ever be the case. What I mean by being ready, is to be able to receive a new perspective and possibly drop any preconceived notions you may have brought with you. In this book you won't find a single thing about losing weight or gaining muscle rapidly.

This book is about looking at health differently, breaking the

cycle of your behaviors, and cutting loose the mindset that got you to where you are in the first place.

True growth requires a certain degree of humility to move forward in a way you haven't before, a starting over if you will. It bruises the ego and can shatter your identity. It can make you want to hide in a cave because you don't recognize what you've let yourself become. If you're not ready for that, then set this book aside for a later day.

You can rest easy, though, that there will not be any brow beating or shaming in this book. But you might get emotional. Actually, I really hope you do, but in a "this is good for me" kind of way. I believe that most people are doing the best they can with the upbringing, resources and information they have been exposed to. However, in order for health and fitness to finally stick, we have to start looking at things from a different angle.

The truth is, you can eat only organic foods, see a doctor every week to run tests, exercise every day, see a therapist, meditate and micromanage your biology with supplements, but something is still going to kill you.

So, let's not get neurotic about this stuff either. Health and fitness are something we integrate into our lives in order to enjoy the things we love even more. It's about living the life we truly want to as long as we can. If we obsess over it, it turns in on itself and becomes an ironic crutch that enables us instead of empowers us.

I really don't know what's going to happen to me when I die. Of course, I have my own personal beliefs, but in the end I really just don't know. I've never been dead before. What I do know is that I'm alive right now, and that's a gift of the most divine privilege. With that being understood, I choose to bet my chips down on this life here and now. The odds of all the things that had to happen in the history of the world in order for me to have been born has been estimated to be upward of 1 in 400 trillion. That means our lives are literally miraculous even from a mathematical sense. I'd be an idiot not to take that as a blessing.

The ultimate display of both intelligence and gratitude for this life we were given is to try our best to *live better and try to die a little slower*.

I don't have answers; I just have experiences and that's what this book is about. Like every teacher, doctor, artist, sanitation worker, supreme court justice, and every other person on this planet, I'm making this *life-stuff* up as I go along. My hope is that there is something about me finding my way through health and fitness that you find useful.

Step 1

AWAKEN

1.

"And you may ask yourself…
Well how did I get here?"

— Talking Heads, Once in A Lifetime

In 1982, I was six years old, and my dad was driving me down Main Street in Dayton, Ohio. I was in the passenger seat (back before there were booster seat laws) and he said, "Eric, do you know what divorce means?". I had a vague idea, because there was a girl in my first-grade class whose parents had just gotten divorced. I remember being very confused about how something like that even worked. Next thing I knew, later that night my mom was crying in the kitchen and my grandparents had arrived from Indianapolis to take my mom and me back with them. To this day, the most vivid memory I have is of my mother and grandfather prying me away from my father. It was slightly painful to even write that paragraph.

My mom and I moved to Indianapolis permanently, and she got a job making $13k a year as a secretary (that's what they called administrative positions back then). Our living arrangements were pretty much what you'd imagine. An apartment with a refrigerator mostly filled with condiments in a somewhat shady neighborhood. My clothes mostly came from garage sales and K-mart. Dinner was mostly hot dogs on stale sandwich bread, or mac and cheese made with water instead of milk.

My mom tried to find affordable daycare for me after school, but there were many days where I came home to an empty apartment. I was a tried and true "latchkey kid" from an early age. Those few hours after school were actually a nightmare for me, starting with the bus ride home. As you might expect from a kid whose life was just completely uprooted, I was sad, scared and reclusive, so I became a target for bullies. I would get picked on during the whole bus ride, and by the time we I got off the bus I was fuming. This resulted in a lot of fights with the neighborhood kids.

And I lost every one of those fights. Every. Single. One.

You know you lost a bus stop fight because when the fight is over you are standing all alone while there are five or six kids standing behind the other guy. The fights weren't brutal, because we were just little kids, but they were definitely traumatic. I bottled them up inside and rarely told anyone about them.

My mom had no idea what to do with me. She tried to get me into sports, probably to toughen me up, but that made things worse because I was absolutely terrible at everything. I struck out every time I was at bat and was as awkward as could be. No one wanted to sit next to me or be my friend, and the coach sure as hell didn't want me to play much. All of this naturally created a need to numb my pain.

As soon as I arrived home after school, I began to take refuge with whatever was in the fridge.

With limited options, I would have to be creative. I usually made a sandwich with some kind of salad dressing on the aforementioned stale bread. I would put away four or five of those sandwiches before my mom got home from work. Needless to say, I gained a lot of weight and became an even bigger target for bullies. Literally.

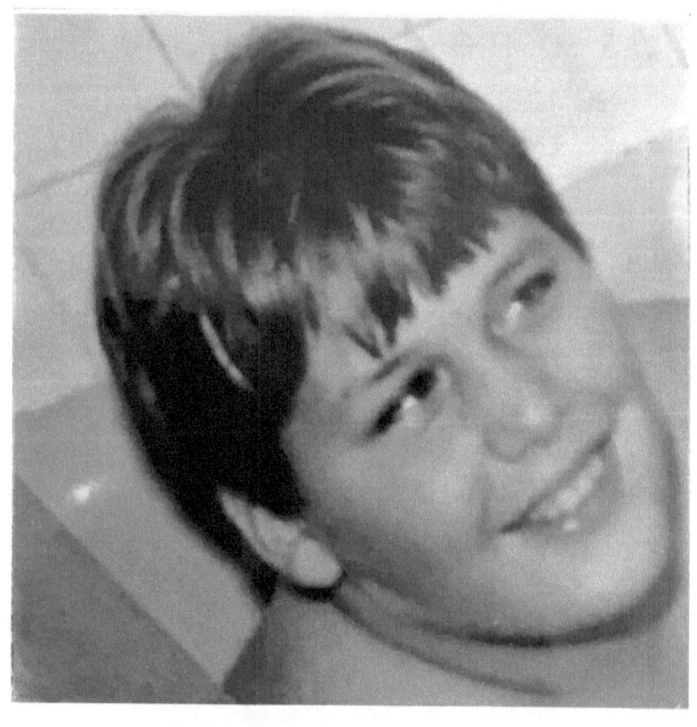

Not exactly sure of my age here, but I'd say I was around 9 years old in this picture.

Over time, my sadness and anxiety turned into a quick trigger for anger, and I retreated from any desire to try and make friends. Somehow, I seemed to always have one quasi-friend which probably kept me from going off the deep end, but I always still felt like a loner. Most days I treated my mom like shit, because I needed a release. Even though It had been my dad who pushed her for a divorce, none of that mattered or crossed my mind. My mom was the most convenient target for my rage, simply because she was there.

What made me even more of a little prick to my mom was I'd sabotage every new relationship she tried to get in with another man. For the record, I love my mom tremendously, and have apologized profusely for who I was to her back then. She worked her ass off, and struggled to give me a life that was safe all while I showed her my contempt. That's the true definition of a mother's love.

And to this day I respect single mothers more than any other species on the planet.

But I digress. One day, my mom brought home a new guy for me to meet, someone from work who she'd been dating for a couple months. I remember him coming over for dinner; my mom had cooked Italian food. I'd started to show some promise in art, and he was very complimentary of some of my work that was hanging on the fridge. In return, I was cautiously warm towards him.

He was only sixteen years older than me and had no kids, so he was a little more fun than some of the other guys my mom had introduced me to. He was also a graduate of Notre Dame and a huge football fan. At age 26, he was still full of energy and youthful drive. He took me out to see movies and get pizza, which for some reason the others didn't. He was a fun guy.

One time he took me out to play catch with a football, and according to him, he came back to the apartment and cried to my mom. I was that bad. Despite what must have been serious reservations towards taking on a basket case of a kid who was already ten years old, this young guy, with his whole life in front of him, became my stepfather. Now, while having a consistent male figure improved my life tenfold, I still didn't make it easy on him either. I was still a traumatized kid, so I was a tyrant when he tried to discipline me and we had countless explosive arguments. Coming from a traumatic childhood himself, coupled with the added stress of integrating into a new step-family, he often coped with alcohol back then. I can't blame him at all.

Needless to say, during my teenage years, fighting and

screaming became a common form of communication at our house.

But some good things started to happen to me too. In 8th grade I grew a lot taller, which thinned me out and slowly gave me a little boost of confidence. Because of my size, I was actually able to play on the football team as a lineman (I sure as hell still couldn't throw, catch or run). This also gave me a little taste of popularity and attention from the girls. Unfortunately, I quickly became addicted to receiving attention from my peers.

Of course, I still hadn't dealt with any of my underlying insecurities and anger, so when my popularity would wane or my status was threatened, my behavior would turn ugly.

I ruined every relationship with girls because of my jealousy and insecurity. In hindsight, I was practically bipolar with my need to show them over-the-top affection, and then do a 180 degree turn into a jealous rage if my girlfriend wanted to do anything other than be with me.

By the time I was a senior in high school, I started dating a girl a couple of years younger than me. The next year, I went away to college in Texas, but tried to stay together with her. I completely wasted a semester love-sick and too afraid to integrate. I came home a few months later with four credit hours (one of them was in archery), hundreds of dollars in unpaid long-distance bills, and a couple of credit cards that I'd maxed out. All I had done the entire time was stay in my room, play video games, and try to call my girlfriend back home.

I returned home to enroll in a local college while we carried on our dysfunctional relationship. We soon decided to raise the stakes and get married. I was only twenty-one at the time, doing terribly in college and racking up some serious debt. I spent money, drank, smoked and ate junk food to fill my void. Eventually I dropped out of college completely, started bartending and doing other crappy jobs I didn't like. My relationship with my wife deteriorated quickly. She wanted to live her life, have fun, and thrive; I wanted to stay home, have her to myself and start getting old. She was completely miserable, and so was I.

Eight months later we filed bankruptcy, and she left me a week after that. She was very smart to do so.

Now as you can imagine, a child of divorce has some serious abandonment issues, and when she walked out and wanted a divorce I was absolutely crushed. For days, I laid on the floor and cried. Every now and then I got up to smoke a cigarette, but that's about it. I was now completely alone, and about eighty pounds overweight (I was bigger than I had ever been). The idea of being single, overweight and unlovable was very heavy.

I started to put anything in my body to numb the pain, and I'd go anywhere with anybody in order to distract me. This was my rock bottom.

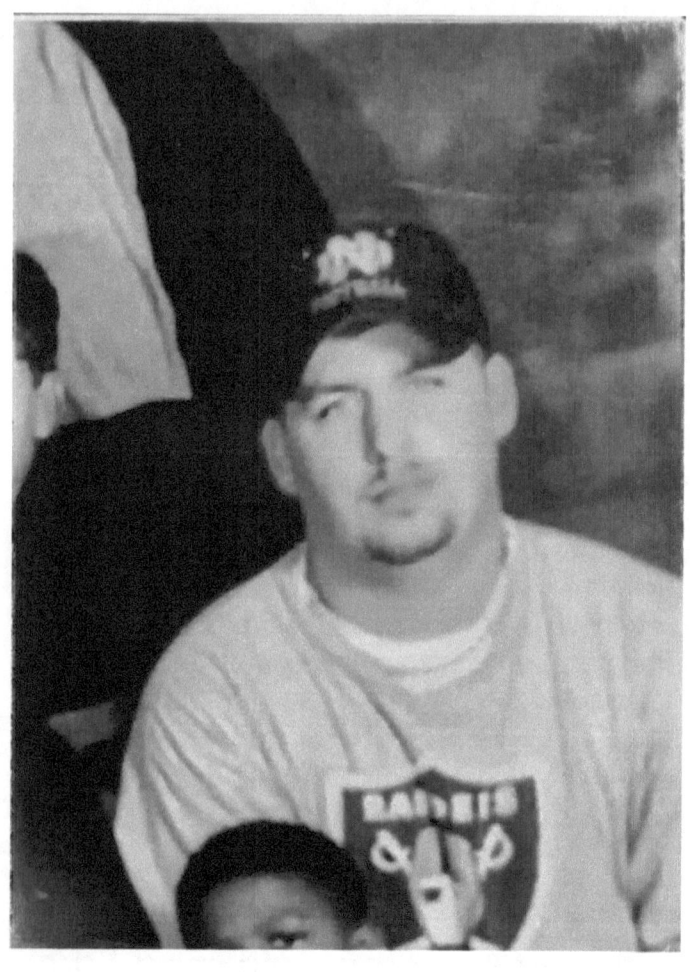

Age 22. I helped coach a youth football team in Lawrence, Indiana. I weighed about 250ish pounds in this picture.

My stepfather was the one who helped pull me out of the darkness though. He came over to my place one day and gave it to me straight. "You need to pick yourself up by the bootstraps", is what I remember the most from that conversation. He must have known there was a lot riding on that pep talk, because for some reason he got through to me that night. In a couple of days, I started to pull myself up and get back in the game of life slowly. I remember I came up with a mantra (before I even knew what a mantra was), and it was, "be the better man". This was my way of reminding myself I needed to improve.

I hated who I'd become, but unfortunately my intentions of "being the better man" were still misplaced. Be better than who???

Looking back, I remember thinking that if I could just elevate myself over others then I would be happy, that I would be climbing. I needed to stand out in a new way. The year that followed consisted of popping diet pills to lose weight, smoking pot with my friends and engaging in philosophical debates all day long. I thought I was opening my mind and exploring a new sense of self. I would engage in argumentative philosophical conversations like a sport, but they were usually egotistically driven, and I only cared about proving how smart I was. That was supposedly filling the void of all the stupid shit I was doing.

Bottom line, I was trying way too hard to impress people, because I had just shown the world that I was a big bankrupt and divorced failure who really didn't have his life together. I started by trying to fix myself on the surface, and trying to change the way I wanted other people to see me. Every other week I was coming up with a big idea that would make me a lot of money or elevate my status in the world, because that's what I thought would neutralize my pain. It was a bad kind of ambition. Driven by a delusional expectation while not doing any of the real work that it takes to change who you are.

However, in hindsight, it still was a very special time. Despite the fact that my daily discipline was mainly self-indulgence, for the first time in my life I was actually thinking differently about things. I was looking to try and make sense of who I was, and more importantly, what I wanted to do with my time on earth. Even though they were naïve and bloated, my desires were still rooted in some form of wanting to change for the better.

Then for some reason, the universe decided to throw me a bone.

Later that year, I got set up on a date with a girl who was seriously out of my league. Denise had just built her first home, had a great job, and was training to qualify for the Boston Marathon. I, on the other hand, was a college dropout, marijuana aficionado with $18 in my checking account (which I was soon to overdraw). During the day I was selling discount furniture, by night I was writing a half-assed screenplay so I could move out to Hollywood and claim my rightful place among the elite. I was also good at eating Taco Bell at 1am, and smoking at least a pack of cigarettes every day. For some reason she still thought she'd give me a chance.

For our first date, I borrowed my stepfather's car to take her to a fancy steakhouse that I couldn't afford. Once again, I was all about trying to impress. I was a little caught off guard when she only ordered a Caesar salad. Apparently, she was a vegetarian, so I was off to a great start. Regardless, we went out a few more times, and I must have made her laugh just the right way because she liked me enough to eventually marry me. I found out much later that what really sold her was my drunk Christmas party dancing skills, and when I acted like a monkey in my underwear. Love is strange.

Denise was the first person I had spent any time with who actually had her head on straight. I was enamored by her. She was basically my first health coach, and simply by being with her I got to observe how mature, responsible people live on a daily basis. Looking back, the most amazing thing about our relationship was that she never tried to change me. I was not a project to her, and she never got upset by my delayed maturity.

She was wise enough to let me develop in my own time.

A couple of years later we had our first child, and like many new parents, I was thrust into a much different idea of what responsibility really means. I was now responsible for how another human being turned out. I had little eyes watching everything I did, and I sure as hell wasn't going to let my children experience anything that resembled my childhood. My dysfunctional baggage was going to end with me.

From that point on I decided I wasn't going to try to be "*The* better man" anymore. I was simply going to be "*A* better man". Playing the long game was now my only reality.

At the time, I was focusing on art and music, but my health, self-doubt, and anxiety were still not in check. I was doing better than I ever had been, but I needed some help. More than twenty years after my parents divorced, I found myself walking into a martial arts academy.

Finally, I was ready to get serious about digging into a part of me that I had been neglecting and running from. It was time to focus and put in the next level of work.

I was scared out of my mind, because all my traumatic childhood memories of fighting with bullies and athletic incompetency were walking in that door with me. When I looked around the room, I saw men, but I truly felt like a boy. For the next few months, I contemplated quitting every single day, but I kept coming back. I simply knew this was something I had to overcome. At any other time in my life I would have quit. I was constantly injured and bruised (including my ego), but I was beginning to feel alive like I never had been before.

What I didn't realize was that I was finally coming into my own maturity and developing a self-awareness like never before. Very slowly, but surely.

My ego was being challenged, my nervous system was being challenged, I was learning how to stay calm under stress, and my mind was becoming clearer.

Something strange was happening, and I was starting to realize that I was capable of living a very different kind of life. Soon I even started running, lifting weights, taking yoga and changing my diet. The better my body was performing, the better my mind and heart were feeling. I was actually taking care of myself for the first time in my life.

I wasn't just getting in shape… I was becoming happier.

After many years, I was beginning to feel capable and maybe worthy of helping others too.

Now, I am completely mesmerized with the body-mind connection, and how self-care affects every aspect of our being. My mental health, parenting style, relationships and my outlook on the entire world has shifted lock step with my physical health.

I am convinced creating healthier people is the best way to make the world a better place, *and this is the hill I am willing to die on*.

In 2013, I started my own business and named it Seva Fitness. Years before, Nicole Brown, an amazing mentor and yoga instructor, introduced me to the idea that taking care of yourself is actually an act of service for those you love. It's a very powerful idea which is supported by Samuel Johnson's quote,

"To preserve health is a moral duty... We can no longer be useful when we are not well."

I named my business "Seva" which is an ancient Sanskrit word that means "to serve", and I have dedicated my professional and personal life to this concept. To make fitness accessible to everyone, and to show what's really at stake if you neglect it.

Our first tagline at Seva was "Make yourself better, make the world better."

Seva Fitness was born from the ashes of dysfunction and failure. I have spent my life on both sides of the self-care fence, and this has allowed me to truly relate to many of my clients' struggles with integrating a self-care routine into their lifestyles. While I still grapple with some of the remnants of my past, I wouldn't trade them for any amount of money. The past is where the healing is, the present is where you will find your true power, and the future is where we unfold into the person we've always had the potential to be.

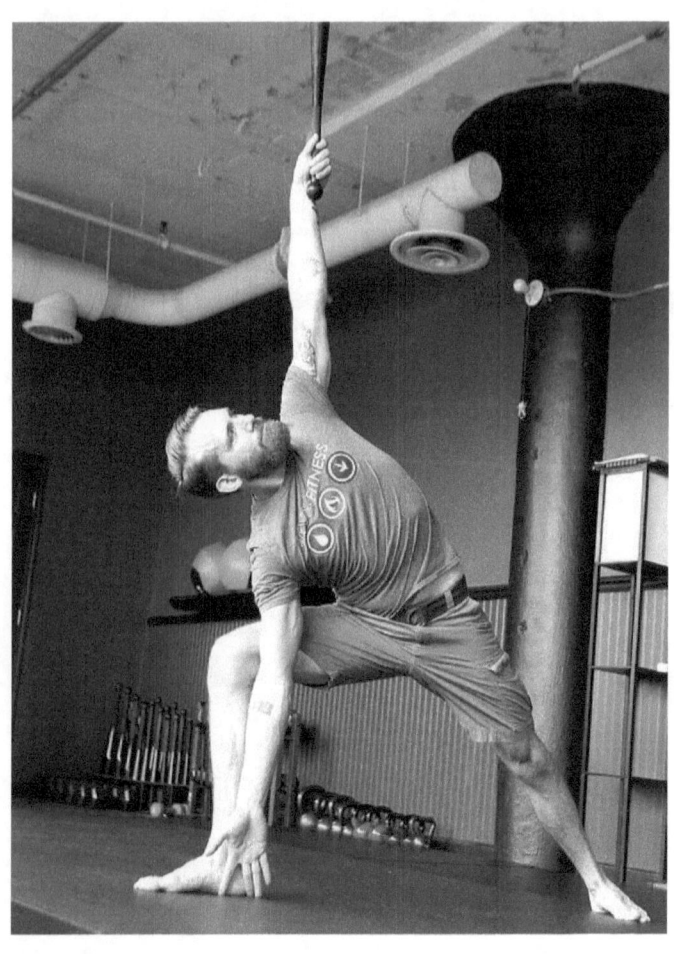

Age 40. 2016

2.

"He who has health, has hope.
He who has hope, has
everything"

— Thomas Carlyle

Perhaps my biggest motivator in all things is
improving my quality of life. If you haven't come to
that conclusion yourself, then you should probably
put this book down. Each one of us gets to define
what 'quality of life' means, but pursuing it is the

reason we go to work and do everything we do. On a base level, making money is a means to keep a roof over our heads, survive the elements and put food in our bellies. But that's merely the *base level* of life quality. I don't want to drop anchor there. Life is not just about getting the bills paid. This life has a lot more to offer, and with a few other considerations we can really make things better for ourselves.

Being human is crazy. Specifically, being human on this side of the twentieth century. If you think about it, we're really just a bunch of mammals that have invented countless ways to keep busy on this big blue orb in the vastness of infinite space. That's a groovy cocktail right there. In our early stages of existence, things were a bit more elementary. By that, I don't mean *easy* - just less complicated. The daily agenda for us humanoids was just to follow our natural instincts and survive. Modern living is obviously a little different, but if we peel back the layers of technology and contemporary comforts that we wrap ourselves in, we still respond to the same natural urges that our ancestors had.

In short, we are still just cavemen, but with smart phones.

Ten thousand years ago, the agricultural revolution shifted most of us out of primal hunter-gatherer survival mode, and onto a trajectory towards civilization as we know it today. With agriculture, we turned to land occupying and wealth-building to make us feel more secure. Since then, this kind of living has created a chain of innovations and technologies that allow us to live much longer, and more comfortably than our predecessors did. The quest for longevity and a life of comforts is merely an extension of our primal hardwiring to survive. But let me say this right upfront...

It's very important not to confuse living a long life with living a *great life*.

Unfortunately, we all can fall into the trap of favoring quantity over quality. Realistically though, longevity isn't even a key indicator of health. Think of it this way, you can own a rusty, piece-of-shit car that is loud, obnoxious and can't do over thirty miles an hour, but seems to last forever. That doesn't mean it's a good car. Our medical model gravitated towards reducing our pains and increasing longevity, because that's what the market demanded. However, we may have unconsciously started to redefine our model of health based on that too. In other words, a *medical model* is not the same as a *health model*.

It's been said before in many ways, but the message rings true: *health is our greatest wealth*. My goal for this book is to get you to understand this truth a little deeper than before. The closer this gets to your root system, the more you'll start making better choices. *Health affects all things holistically*; you can bet on it! When the spiritual leader, the Dalai Lama was asked what surprised him most about humanity, he said, "Man. Because he sacrifices his health in order to make money. Then he sacrifices money to recuperate his health. And then he is so anxious about the future that he does not enjoy the present; the result being that he does not live in the present or the future; he lives as if he's never going to die, and then dies having never really lived."

That is not the mindset of someone who is rich in health.

Health is human functionality at its highest level; physical, mental and emotional.

In my business as a health coach and trainer, a lot of people come to try and recover what they've neglected and lost in their youth. You might be thinking, "Everyone is going to get old and break down". Yes, you are one hundred percent correct. Can we recover everything? We cannot, but the aging process can be dramatically slowed by lifestyle choices.

The rate at which we are aging in this culture is not normal.

What's very frustrating for a lot of people, is that they *know* how important health is, but they just can't escape their "responsibilities". It's so easy to get wrapped up in the immediacies of life and forget to see the big picture...

But your health is your main responsibility. Without it you die, literally. Neglecting your health is inviting disease and deterioration to move into your system without a fight.

On the flip side, prioritizing your health will ultimately make you more effective and even mentally healthier in every aspect of your life.

You can make time and allocate resources for exercise, eating better, and your mental health; or you can make time and devote resources for injuries, illness and feeling hopeless. Either way there's going to be sacrifice.

All humans, including myself, spend a lot of mental bandwidth on things that aren't really important at all just because of their proximity. It's actually in our hardwiring. I learned a very interesting principle while studying Brazilian Jiu Jitsu with Professor Jared Jessup, an amazing mentor of mine. He wanted to show me how "pressure dictates attention" on a deep psychological level for humans. He explained that we're wired to be hyper-focused on what's giving us stress at any given moment in our lives, but if we're not careful it will distract us from the real solutions.

When we're young (and our health isn't much of a concern), we're wrapped up in the busy-ness of life. Busy-ness soon turns into business, then career building, then taking care of family and financial responsibilities, responding to emails, and before we know it, we're slowly being choked by the immediacies of each day.

During a Jiu Jitsu lesson, Jared taught me how this principle shows up even in a violent situation. The lesson that day was to learn how to defend myself if someone were to choke me with their hands. Jared stood in front of me, placed his hands around the front my neck and started to squeeze (don't worry, this dude had Jedi sensitivity), and then asked, "What do you think you should do?". Of course, because of the pressure on my neck, all I could think about was grabbing his hands, since that was where the pressure was coming from.

That's what people are wired to do.

However, he was stronger than me and I was running out of air, which made my efforts less and less effective. Finally, he knew I had realized the degree of my incompetence, and showed me how my solution was right under my feet. Literally.

He demonstrated by taking my place as the victim. As I started to choke him, he simply took one big step back and bent his knees in a widened stance so that he was solidly planted into the floor. He termed it "getting in base". Then, he folded at the waist and ducked under my hands effortlessly.

44

Instead of getting caught up in defending against my hands and wasting a lot of his energy, he positioned himself in a strong foundation and used the full weight and strength of his body to break through the two tiny thumbs that were causing all the pressure on his throat. In that single move, he showed me that by focusing on the right things, I can get a lot more done with much less effort.

Health is that foundation in our lives that makes us get more done with less effort. Like my lack of knowledge in self-defense at that time, I believe that humans have major gaps in knowledge when it comes to understanding the true value and potency of personal health. In a rapid-fire culture, we don't always think about how productive it is to move towards biological progress instead of passive decline.

We forget, we're inhabiting the only body and brain we're ever going to have. We don't get to trade in our vehicle.

There's a reason why high performers value their workouts, diets and developmental routines above all else.

Entrepreneurs, executives, musicians, athletes - virtually anyone who takes their daily performance seriously understands the true value and potency of health. And they want more of it!

Unfortunately, the people who need to shift their focus towards their health the most, are those fighting on the front lines of everyday life. They are our teachers, parents, caregivers, soldiers, leaders, volunteers and anyone who serves others. They are much more valuable to us if they're healthy and thriving, instead of exhausted and sick.

Out of curiosity I wanted to see what the first thing that popped up on google would be if I typed in "the definition of health". The result was, *Health: The state of being free from illness or injury.* Culturally speaking that sounds about right, but I take issue with it. What's wrong with that, you might ask? First of all, this definition presents health as a *lack* of something. That's like saying that because you don't have a bankruptcy on your record, you're doing great financially. Health is like energy economics.

Health is energy, and acts a lot like money. *We need energy for everything we do*, so health is an asset we need to acquire.

Have you ever had a day when your energy bank was low? Of course you have, and on those days, everything is a little bit harder. Now think about how a steady decline in your health could slowly creep up on you, and makes your everyday responsibilities more difficult.

Eventually, this will bring you to the point of slowly withdrawing from things you love, because you just can't handle life like you used to.

This doesn't just affect us as we get older though. When my son was on his school's academic team, the teachers and parents would bring in food for them to eat 60 to 90 minutes before their match. Don't get me wrong, their intentions were good, but all of the snacks consisted of starchy simple carbohydrates and/or sugar. The problem was, no one understood how much nutrition affects human performance, and like clockwork I would watch the kids' energy levels crash about 45 minutes later. Sometimes even right in the middle of their match. If they had simply waited to feed them until twenty minutes before their match, even the junk food could've been used productively as an energy boost. Of course, I tried to explain this to the powers that be, but my concerns fell on deaf ears.

We have no reservations about why top athletes are on focused diet programs to fuel their bodies properly, but for some reason we disregard the need to protect and maintain the energy levels in our everyday lives. Performance is performance.

If you like to work twice as hard to get half as much done, then don't worry about this health stuff. But don't bullshit yourself, the human machine can only perform to the degree that it's taken care of, so don't expect too much out of life either. You can treat your body like a luxury sports car, keeping it finely tuned and using good fuel, or you can treat it like an unappreciated used car that was given to you for free. In the end, it will perform according to how it's been maintained and invested in.

3.

"Life doesn't get easier or more forgiving, we get stronger and more resilient."

- Steve Maraboli

I'm not going to lie. These next couple of chapters might touch a few exposed nerves and even shake up some emotions. They are definitely going to be centered around being uncomfortable.

Unfortunately, if we spend too long neglecting our health, having ice water dumped on us while we sleep can be the only prescription that works. I can feel some of you squirming in your chair already, and I get it. There are plenty of things in life that can make you feel like life is beating you down enough already. You may be putting up with soul sucking corporate bullshit, an unsupportive spouse, children who are seriously struggling, or maybe you just walk around with the heaviness of trauma and/or shame. There are very few of us that haven't been through some kind of fiery hell that we call our own.

None of that is enough to warrant throwing in the towel. On the contrary, it means you need to get your head in the game even more and start performing better.

If you're going to tackle getting healthy, and making it stick, you're going to have to handle things a little different this time. Look through a different lens, and maybe dig a little deeper in the emotional suitcase you've been carrying. It may be necessary to question things about your upbringing and the cultural values you embrace. All of your answers are there to be found, but usually we are the ones refusing to pull back the curtain.

In the fitness industry there is a saying called "embracing the suck". It can have a few different connotations, but mostly it means that the discomfort you are going to go through will be medicinal. Eventually it will be life giving and not life draining, but at first, it's going to be a bitter, jagged pill to the ego and body. If you can keep the medicine down though, it will end up being a Mario-Power-Up mushroom to your body and soul. However, in order to really be able to embrace this initial suck phase, it's critically important to know a little more about the hidden value of stress.

Our culture in the West has been the victor of some of humanity's most amazing struggles and the benefactor of its spoils. Historically I know there is a lot more nuance to how we got here, but the point I'm trying to make is that we are a civilization that was forged through struggle. Something very interesting has happened since WWII. After the Greatest Generation won the greatest battle, they came back and built an amazing infrastructure for the next generations.

New innovations and technologies would help keep us on top in the world of commerce and civilization building. These new innovations and technologies were often designed to make our lives easier and more comfortable. What we didn't realize was that there were going to be some serious unwanted side effect to all that comfort.

The world of innovation created less of a need to be physically active.

Efficient business systems were being built, and the increase in office jobs quickly thrust us into a more sedentary lifestyle.

Human beings are stress-adaptation machines. It's one of our greatest strengths as a species. If it wasn't for the adaptations our ancestors made for the past two million years, none of us would be here. For our ancestors, the constant threat of survival was a stress that kept them active and sharp. As modern humans, we very rarely experience that same kind of stress, and to be honest that's probably a good thing. But that doesn't take away the fact that…

Our bodies and minds were designed to move and take on physical stress. Without an appropriate dosage of stress, we become weak, dull and imbalanced throughout our entire system.

Stress resiliency is often misunderstood at best and under-valued at worst. For many people the kind of mental stress that they experience throughout the day can be toxic and deteriorative. This can make the entire idea of stress a negative thing in the minds of most people. Typically, we aren't taught how to handle stress in a healthy way. We are told to push it down and tough it out, but that's not how stress resiliency works.

The ability to bounce back from stress and use it positively is a more important skill than trying to resist or escape it.

Stress resilience is something some people figure out, and some people don't. No matter what, it's something none of us can learn to thrive without.

Stress is a constant part of life, and not all stresses are equal. In fact, in terms of creating health and vitality, stress is our number one ally.

The key to making stress work for you lies in the dosage. It needs to be *appropriate*, and that is different for everyone. Stress that happens too rapidly--or too intensely--will cause a negative adaptation. Things like seeing a person die suddenly, a loud noise next to your open ear, or falling off a tall ladder can cause either mental or physical traumas, both of which are negative stress adaptations. Trauma is one end of the negative stress pendulum.

When it comes to negative stress, too much is also the same thing as too little.

Things like sitting too long, becoming socially reclusive, having a broken arm in a cast or always using your GPS instead of paying attention to your orientation are all ways the brain and body can begin to atrophy. This means the stress is insufficient for growth. Most of us can recognize the places in our lives where stress feels too high and, likewise, where the stress feels too low. When we spend our day at work where we might be sitting in a chair (insufficient physical stress), but yet simultaneously having high emotional or mental stress, that is a perfect storm for disease and dysfunction, either mental, physical, or even both.

But right in the middle of the stress pendulum is a magical little goldilocks zone of positive stress called eustress. This is where health and *even happiness* can be found.

Modern humans commonly swing their pendulum from high levels of stress to low levels of stress in their daily cycle. It's completely normal, as it's the body's way of finding balance called homeostasis. The size of the swing, however, can be destructive to the human machine if taken to extremes for too long. If you work all day under consistent high levels of stress, and then go home and collapse and self-medicate, it's like driving your car 90 miles an hour and slamming the brakes all the time. Yeah, you'll get places that way, but your vehicle will pay for it and it won't be a very enjoyable ride. Getting away from the extremes of stress is where exercise comes into play.

Exercise, in its simplest form, *is self-induced stress that is designed to create positive adaptations in the body when done appropriately*. Healthy exercise helps keep our system in the positive stress zone throughout the day, and actually teaches our body, mind and nervous system to deal with stress in a positive way. When exercise and movement are lacking in our human machine, a few big problems start to occur.

First of all, it's important to know that the mental and emotional stress we have throughout our day is released in the form of a chemical cocktail which goes into the tissue throughout our body. Sometimes it can even be felt in areas like your neck, shoulders, back, hands or may even present itself in the form of a headache. These are just a few of the more obvious ones. What's critical to know is that…

Without strenuous movement the stress deposits in your body don't get broken up. Over time the stress build-up becomes very toxic bio-chemically causing a cascade of stress-related diseases.

How mental stress affects the body is a simple concept but can be easily overlooked as we spend most of our perceived reality in our heads. One of the most important ideas that I want to get my clients to realize is *movement is life!*

We have to move our bodies in order to achieve any higher quality of life. It's a very elemental point. Life is animated, and things that are diseased or dying move less.

Think of it this way, you can't drink water from a stagnant puddle. Without movement and circulation there is no purification. This is exactly what is going on with our biochemistry internally, but this is just the beginning.

Without targeted movements to areas of the body heavily affected by stress, the stress deposited into our tissue begins to harden. Not only does this hardening tissue affect our ranges of motion, it also begins to pull our bones out of alignment. This coupled with the adaptations from prolonged sitting cause our bone structure and body mechanics to become critically dysfunctional. It will even affect the way we look. There's a reason athletes look upright and confident while desk jockeys can often look frumpy and apathetic. It's not the muscles and leaner bodies, it's their bone structure coupled with the vitality in their veins.

As your bone structure becomes more misaligned, a cascade of other issues and symptoms are certain to follow. First, you may notice mild to moderate aches and pains in your joints. Since your bone structure is constantly being pulled, there will naturally be a sense of prolonged strain and tension that will be hard to get relief from. Since chronic strain to the skeletal structure takes a toll on your circulation (think of what happens when you kink a garden hose), next usually comes an increase in lethargy and compromised moods. In addition, everyday things like walking, going up stairs, and mowing the yard take a larger toll on you than they used to because your body is working against itself mechanically.

That decrease in performance is not from aging, it's from neglect.

Finally come the injuries, which often happen when you are trying to get back into the habit of exercise, or when you are doing something simple like yard work. Hopefully the injury isn't too serious, but often times it's something that can keep you from doing the things you love, or would like to do someday.

Piggy-backing off the cascade of structural and physical issues comes even more mental and emotional stress.

Witnessing your own physical decline isn't something that makes anyone feel better. It can even change your world view and cause strain on your relationships.

I've never met someone who loves feeling weakened. Now, do people learn to cope with those feelings? All the time. But my point is, you don't have to lose your strength, mobility, and other physical attributes prematurely. *The majority of our deterioration is lifestyle-induced and accelerated.*

When we put our health and self-care in its rightful place, we avoid a lot of unnecessary discomfort (the bad kind). By trying to avoid the positive stress associated with exercise and behavior change, we are essentially saying we'd rather have the perpetual negative stress of increasing chronic pains, handicaps, increased medical expenses, illness and disease, not to mention the emotional toll of self-doubt, shame, rapid aging and diminished competency.

Make no mistake, this is the trajectory of anyone who neglects their health. If you can't change your routine of comfort, ironically, it will break you.

"It is difficult to free fools from the chains they revere." – Voltaire

Don't be a fool. I promise neglecting your health is way more difficult than the discomfort of exercise and using a little restraint in your life. Don't worry, I'm going to help you get started.

If you are truly ready to change, it's going to require some humility, and perhaps some brutal honesty. It's time to dig down to the roots of your behaviors and what's really holding you back. If you can do that, your courage will always be rewarded with hope and growth.

When you're ready, turn the page.

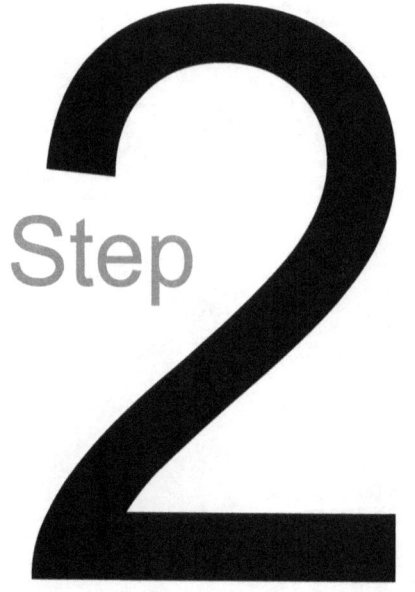

Step

2

ALIGN

4.

"Once we accept our limits, we go beyond them."

— Albert Einstein

Inscribed at The Temple of Apollo at Delphi is the Ancient Greek aphorism, *Gnothi seauton.* It translates into the phrase, "know thyself." It's an idea that Socrates expanded by proclaiming, "the unexamined life is not worth living." Personally, I would take that even a step further and say not actively trying to understand yourself better, and why you do the things you do, makes life more difficult than it needs to be.

When I found myself divorced, bankrupt and overweight I looked at myself in the mirror. All I saw was a completely unlovable, overweight, undisciplined sack of shit.

Now, while my therapist may have thought I was being a little too hard on myself, I think it was one of the most important moments in my life. I hated who I had become, and I was finally ready to admit it.

Many of the traumas in my life that made me so insecure were not my fault, but it was my responsibility to figure out who I was going to become from that point on. I had been lying to myself and others for years trying to make people think I was something that I wasn't, and now I couldn't lie any more. I was done with it. I was ready to start from scratch and rebuild.

I have been an addict since I was seven years old. My first addiction was food, then nicotine, throw in some excessive behaviors with weed, sex, porn, sleep…whatever I could use to numb my pain and not face the discomfort of my own feelings has been fair game at one point or another. Hell, I still chew gum like a fiend when I get restless, stay hyper-productive and can even treat exercise excessively sometimes. Like I said, I am still climbing my own mountain.

When I was truly spiraling downward, I was missing one critical element: self-awareness. It wasn't until I started to look at myself with a little more curiosity and a little less judgment, that I started to get a foothold on my behaviors.

At some point we all need to look into a mirror with both brutal honesty and radical compassion in order to change. Without brutal honesty we will never know where we are really starting from, and without radical compassion we will never realize how human our unwanted behaviors really were.

When the playing field finally was leveled, I started to believe I could make some headway. By allowing myself that degree of honesty I was able to finally take ownership of my life and start moving forward instead of being passive. Then, by understanding there was a primal psychology to my behaviors, I realized my failure wasn't just about me being a weak or broken person. My insecurities finally were easing up, and my hopes were authentically rising. Author, playwright and actress Tina Lifford completely nailed it when she said,

"When you know yourself, you are empowered. When you accept yourself, you are invincible."

Trust me, you are not broken. You are just doing what humans do when they've been exposed to what you have. All the variables in your life so far have intersected with your human hardwiring to make you who you are right this very second.

One of the most important things I ever learned was another lesson that came from training in martial arts. I learned that it isn't our thoughts that are the root of our behavior, it's our nervous system that's driving the bus. In other words, our thoughts come from the stimulation our nervous system receives. Without training, our primal *reflexive* hardwiring makes us do what we do, and it just shows up in subtle ways in modern life. All humans are susceptible to this. For people who deal with trauma and addiction, this knowledge is incredibly important to understand.

Our first directive as humans is to survive against threats. All our behaviors can be seen as an extension of that order.

That is to say, if you were a computer, the first line of code that would be written into your programming would be "Survive". All other functions and behaviors would in some way be based off of this.

We were given the gift of *fight-flight-freeze* in order to deal with threats. You wouldn't be alive without it. The problem is that is a short-term survival model and not a long-term wellness model. It is reflexive and not responsive. We have to learn how to write new lines of code so we can move from *survive to thrive*. Naturally, before we start to reprogram our behaviors, we have to be in touch with the source of our unwanted, reflexive, and out-of-control behaviors. Then we have to begin to accept them. Remember, you are not broken. You are just doing what humans do.

All day long, your nervous system is collecting data and interpreting the threats in your environment.

To your nervous system, just about everything is a threat. It can't tell the difference between a legitimate threat and a perceived

threat; it only measures the intensity and proximity.

Even the tiniest interruptions - like a text message notification - create a subconscious impulse that the body receives and decides how to respond to. Likewise, being cut off in traffic, being interrupted in the middle of something important, navigating through crowds of people, facing deadlines, watching something intense on TV, being confronted on social media about your beliefs, all of these can serve as a threat to your sense of self. In turn your body releases a stress cocktail that elevates your system to prepare for confrontation. Depending on the size of the threat, you'll experience a proportionate dump of adrenaline that provides a burst of energy, strength or even rage in order to get through the threat.

This even plays out in your everyday personality and moods. For example, if you're on a low-stress family vacation, you may be very agreeable and able to brush off the smaller unwanted behaviors that pop up with your kids. But after a very long and stressful day at work, you'll be more likely to blow up at your kid for leaving a sock on the floor. Then we can get caught in a loop where our beliefs and values justify our reflexive behaviors, and at that point we find ourselves in arrested development, all which all essentially stemmed from a lack of awareness of our basic human survival nature.

Being reflexive or reactive has merit in an acute situation where a threat is serious and immediate. However, in everyday life it just makes you a high-strung and unskilled asshole. In martial arts… White belts *react*, black belts *respond*.

Once we begin to see how this primal behavior model still is alive and strong in our modern lives, we get a better understanding of our road ahead and the true nature of our obstacles. To our nervous system, seeking comfort is the same as seeking security which checks off our survival box. This is why addictions, or any comforting behaviors that are repeated daily, can be so hard to break away from. Even though we know they are hurting us, on an unconscious level they are satisfying our most prime directive. *Comfort equals stability. Stability equals survival.*

While being comfortable in today's world makes us feel safe and stabilized, it also leads to passivity in many ways. Physically and mentally this actually makes us weaker. Health and fitness are about making you a more resilient human being for the long haul, as opposed to becoming fragile. Author, influencer, and one of my favorite people of all time Scott Sonnon used to tell us,

"Life comforts the disciplined and disciplines the comfortable."

Bottom line, there is no health, growth or stability without discomfort. Period. While that may be hard to accept, it's true nonetheless. Ultimately, creating a healthy lifestyle becomes an act of systematically picking uncomfortable things to introduce into your life.

Incorporating exercise and healthy eating into your life is

probably never going to be easy or convenient. That's one of the things that makes it so valuable. The same goes for saving money and building wealth.

While all this is much easier to understand intellectually, the real difficulty is always in applying it. We have the tendency to think applying discomfort in our lives is largely a matter of willpower. In my experience, I would say that willpower is a much smaller part of the equation than most people realize.

What's usually most important is the delayering of ignorance and the part of our ego that misguides us. Another one of my brilliant coaches Alberto Gallazzi, pointed out that our main job was to get clients to realize their "Point A". What he meant was, everyone knows their "Point B", or where they want to go. However, without really knowing (and accepting) where their Point A is, they are wandering aimlessly with useless directions.

Most of us really have a hard time objectively seeing where we are starting from, but the ones that do take off very quickly. Sometimes you have to take a step back in order to take 1000 steps forward.

What follows next are what I call the *5 Alignments*. It's important to realize that these alignments are not static, they are dynamic. Every person's experience with them will be different and personal. They can seem to almost change their meaning completely, and even drop out of the sky like an asteroid unexpectedly into your life. Each one is as necessary as the others, and while you must *actively* pursue them, they often will unfold in their own time.

If you are willing to pursue them, no matter the pace, you will feel like you are moving in a direction that makes you feel better in virtually every area of your life. They are perennial truths that can be used in many areas besides health and fitness.

THE FIVE ALIGNMENTS

1. Realize the Emergency
2. Declare your Worth
3. Be the Student
4. Turn "Why" into "How"
5. Make it Fit

Alignment 1: Realize the Emergency

Hopefully by now I've been making the argument well enough that you are realizing that neglecting your health is an absolutely terrible idea, if not one of the worst ideas ever. The price to pay for neglecting it far outweighs the slight discomforts and inconveniences of healthier behaviors. Not only is necessity the mother of all invention, it is also the mother of all momentum.

Sometimes not having a choice is the best thing that can ever happen to us. All of the energy and anxiety of decision making, resource gathering and timing is washed away by the immediacy of the situation.

If you were just in a serious car accident, you aren't going to worry about, or even ask, how much the ambulance ride is going to cost. You are just going to let them load you up and go. You will figure out how to pay the bill later, because action is required now!

Let's get one thing clear: your days left on Earth are officially fucking numbered.

Sorry, not sorry about the language. That statement is as real as it gets. Refusing to spend a little effort towards adding health in your life is the same as pressing on the accelerator to the grave. Take your foot off the gas NOW!

A conversation that I surprisingly still have to have often, is telling people that it's NOT their doctor who is responsible for their health. We have gotten so wrapped up in the idea that when my body breaks down or has an issue, I go to the doctor and they make me better. Yes, this is what doctors are great at, making you feel better.

However, this kind of thinking is like saying you believe a sports

team can win by only playing defense. Your everyday healthy behaviors are what puts points on the board and keeps you out of the doctor's office. Learn to play some offense, because YOU are responsible for your health.

Literally, just two hours ago, I had a conversation with someone close to me that I had been begging to see a chiropractor for years. Finally, after visiting, they were amazed by how much better they were feeling on a daily basis. Happy for them of course, I continued to explain to them, "Now that the chiropractor has improved your spinal alignment, you should begin to work on your core strength so you can hold the alignment in place."

After saying this, the look in their eye might suggest I tried to punch them in the face. Immediately they resisted the idea saying, "Well isn't that what the chiropractor is supposed to be doing?" To which I responded, "It's a temporary adjustment. If you make your core and midline muscles stronger, your spine will remain healthier longer." This interaction summed up exactly the amount of responsibility a lot of us take away from ourselves and try to give to our doctors when it comes to our own health. If you get knee surgery, but don't take the steps to strengthen the system around it, you will still always have a weak knee.

As dramatic and unnerving as it may sound, every decision we make ultimately is making us stronger or weaker. To be passive about your health constitutes a serious lack of intelligence, delusion or ignorance. As much as that is not a nice thing to say, it absolutely has to be realized. To reject, argue or delay it is at your own peril. The sooner you swallow that pill the better. Get in the ambulance, because your declining health is an emergency.

Alignment 2: Declare Your Worth

My grandmother was a saxophone player, and when she died, I inherited her saxophone. A few years later, I decided I might try to learn and play it, so I took it to a music store to get it cleaned up and such. When I went to pick it up, the guy at the shop came out and said, "Do you know what you have here?" Come to find out, it was a rare kind of saxophone and was worth a lot more than I expected. To me, it was just an old instrument that belonged to my grandmother, but to people that knew better, it was much more than that.

Understanding something's value can be very tricky, especially when it comes to declaring our own.

The most painful thing that happens in my coaching sessions is having to convince people that they are worthy of devoting time and resources for taking care of themselves.

I truly don't want to imagine some of the emotional neglect many of these people have had in their lives in order to come to a place where they think self-care is not something they deserve. Obviously, in the most extreme cases, a mental health professional is needed to unwind the irrationality behind this deteriorative logic and get to the source. However, some of us just need a wake-up call.

There are so many ways that we self-sabotage ourselves, but maybe none more than in the realm of declaring self-worth. For the most part, I either see people who have a hyper-inflated sense of themselves, or people who really aren't even thinking about it at all. Probably the most unpopular things I tell people is (another hard truth alert) is:

"Self-care equals self-respect."

That's a very hard idea to accept in a culture where, statistically speaking, most people are unhealthy due to lifestyle choices. Regardless, the logic is sound. We take care of the things we truly respect. If for some reason cars cost 4x what they do now, and we couldn't trade our cars in for 20 years, imagine how different we would treat them.

It turns out my grandmother's saxophone was worth a couple thousand dollars. If I would've put it up for sale on the internet for $150, that's exactly what I would've been paid. Not a penny more. I declared it's worth, and that's what I would've gotten: Just $150. So many of us are doing the same thing and under-valuing ourselves!

If you aren't getting "paid" by life what you think you're worth, then it's because you priced yourself too low.

If you're a parent, think about how much you are worth to your child. Even if you're not a parent, you are somebody else's child. What would your parents think of the way you take care of yourself? How much are you worth to them? What about your spouse, or even your pet?

If you're reading this book, it's probably time to re-evaluate what you are telling yourself you're worth.

Alignment 3: Be the Student

There's an old story of a scholar who was seeking to learn from a great master that lived in a distant village. After traveling for many days, the scholar finally arrived at the village and found the master. Immediately, the scholar wanted to demonstrate his intellect and share his opinions on important matters. The scholar talked on and on for many minutes. Calmly, the master invited the scholar for tea. The scholar continued to talk as the master poured the tea. When the cup was full, the master just kept pouring. The scholar said to the master, "Stop! Don't you realize the cup is already full?" The master replies, "Yes, it is just like your mind. Come back to me when you have emptied your cup."

Humility is very functional, especially in regard to learning. However, we forget this basic virtue when we are overpowered by the need to be seen as competent.

It's amazing how many people come into my office for the first time and spend a significant amount of time telling me how much they already know and have done before. This usually comes from some kind of previous successful attempt at weight loss. In the age of excess information, a lot of people think they have some built-in expertise in nutrition, exercise science and even behavioral psychology. And while you don't necessarily have to have a degree in those fields to be successful in them, you do need to have some experience with creating, but most importantly maintaining results.

Another hard truth alert…

If you really knew what you were doing, you wouldn't be failing at it.

Yes, in the end we could probably distill getting back into shape down to a few main principles. But it takes years and countless hours of training to learn how to put them into practice and outsmart yourself from self -sabotage. The human body is a very sophisticated machine, and each one of them comes with its own unique issues and imbalances. Everybody is an experiment of one. Investing in professional help is an important step to getting off on the right foot. Remember, this is not just about willpower.

One of the first obstacles to get through is your own ego and blind spots. Once you "get over yourself" the hill actually starts to slope downward and the speed of learning greatly increases. Getting assistance from knowledgeable people can give you a perspective you've never seen before and can take years off your learning curve. Asking for help is a very hard thing for a lot of people to do. In our minds we think it is some kind of admission of failure on our part.

In reality, asking for help is one of the ultimate displays of courage and a promise to ourselves that we are truly serious about making a change this time.

This is also why prayer can be such a transformational practice for people. The act of humbling oneself to ask for help or guidance is something very tangible and powerful in terms of personal development. Even if no one was listening on the other end, it would still be productive at chipping away at the destructive side of pride and ego. Asking for help aligns us not only with the reality of our imperfect humanness, but also allows us to receive support that will ultimately strengthen us during a very tough climb.

In the end, the honesty required in this step ultimately creates a huge relief and lifts a large weight off your shoulders.

We spend ridiculous amount of energy putting on a façade of competency in our daily lives.

The faster you can get comfortable with hard truths on this journey, the faster you will make progress, because...

Clarity equals energy.

You are not expected to be good at everything. Plus, everyone likes someone that is truly willing to help themselves and take on the role as student. It's a positive and innocent energy that's a pleasure to be around, and a breath of fresh air. You will find friends and allies fast if you take on the role of a student.

Growing up, I didn't develop much of any athleticism at all until maybe 8th or 9th grade, and the only reason I had some then was because I hit a huge growth spurt. Being a little taller than everyone else for a couple years allowed me to have a slightly more positive experience with my physicality, but I was still very clumsy. It wasn't until I was 30 years old, when my Jiu Jitsu and yoga instructors started showing me *how* my body actually works, that things started to click. Because they were good teachers, they showed me the mechanics piece by piece, and allowed me to develop at an unscheduled pace. For this reason, I was able to achieve a higher degree of physical competency for the first time in my life.

Great teachers and coaches teach us that "everything can be a learned skill".

We don't tend to think of physical attributes as something learned, but I promise you they are. Things like strength, focus, resilience under stress, flexibility, relaxation and other attributes are things that I actually learned (and still learning) how to do. Not only are those things physical attributes, but they are very important *life skills*.

Take a second and ask yourself this simple but very important question,

"If I gave myself enough time, and could break things down into small enough steps, is there anything I couldn't learn?"

In that question lies much of our salvation for change, and the seed of our future confidence. Generally, we don't give ourselves permission to 1.) Be a student, and 2.) Learn at a pace that works best for us.

If you are struggling with making health and fitness stick in your life, then maybe it's time you finally decide to be a student. I promise, *health is a learned skill.* So many times, we cripple ourselves from the very start with unrealistic expectations of success and/or a pressurized timeline that was pulled out of the air completely at random. If you stop watching your weight, and start watching your health you might find the weight falls off easier than it ever has before. Maybe not quite as fast as a fad diet, but definitely more permanent. Then, with a little guidance, you can *learn* how to exercise a greater degree of self-control. Then you can *learn* how to embrace discomfort and enjoy exercise. Most importantly, you can *learn* how to make all of it work for you in the context of your life. Commit to becoming a student for life, and claim your superpower. Live and *learn*.

Alignment 4: Turn "Why" Into "How"

Humans can be motivated and inspired by beautiful things, but we are actually more strongly motivated by the need to numb our pain. This quest for anesthesia looks like anything from self-medicating, addiction, ambition, or staying constantly distracted. The last and most unusual path taken is to face your pain head on. Your emotional pains of the past are usually the wall that stands in between you and the person you deserve to be.

To be clear, everyone deserves health and happiness. However, not everyone earns it.

Quick Assignment:

Make a list of the five things that hurt or embarrassed you the most in your life. Leave a few blank spaces under each entry.

Don't really overthink it. It will probably be the first five things you can think of. Chances are a lot of them happened when we were kids and young adults, so they might seem silly or trivial when you write them down.

Then ask yourself and write underneath:

"How did I bounce back from this? What did I do to protect myself from it happening again? Did I change myself or my personality in some way? Did I take on a new behavior or identity?"

This simple but powerful little exercise has potential to be a great start on your emotional blueprint. It's what makes you who you are, and shows why you live your life the way you do. Of course, it will take some time to unpack all the ways these moments got you to where you are, but you were brave and made a powerful step just by doing the exercise. It might even give you enough courage to go talk to someone who can help you navigate it better.

Becoming able and willing to sit with your pain from the past in a *non-judgmental* way is one of the most important things you can ever do. It is essential for forward progress.

Like an engine, we need to produce emotional heat for horsepower. The kind of power you need for this journey during its low points (and there will be plenty) is not going to come from cold, rational deduction of statistics. This is where the "Why" becomes the "How". You have to be able to quickly identify the reasons you want to grow, and essentially that is to overcome your pain in a long-term way.

After my divorce and bankruptcy, I was mainly fueled by the residue of shame and the fear of living a life unrealized. I was angry with myself and scared that I would be alone in the future. Truth is, fear and shame are quick burning fuels. They act a lot like kindling as they don't typically last very long, but can still be useful to get things started. First things always need to come first, and right now you need to ignite your fire.

I'm not really a snob about what gets you initially motivated, as long as it gets you moving. Don't get me wrong, I think the cleanest and most powerful fuel comes from a passion for serving others and a healthy sense of self-love, but it usually doesn't start there.

Things like fear and self-disgust are still energy, and they can be transformed and purified along the way. Energy is like money; it can be spent on good things or bad things, but it is inherently a neutral resource.

Naturally, as more health and vitality get in your veins, it begins to shape your world view and self-worth more positively. You will find that original energy of self-disgust transforms into something much more beneficial and longer lasting.

Once you have the fire going, it has to be tended to. *It's easy to smother the flame if you're too aggressive.* Remember, a fire requires air. It has to breathe. This is another reason why you can't be fueled mainly by your dark side. It's good for igniting your fire, but not for keeping it going. Your "Why" will need to evolve into a deeper sense of purpose.

Without a deeper purpose, there is no hope for permanent change. This is why superficial reasons for taking care of yourself always bring temporary results. Losing weight simply to look better in your bathing suit is a surface-level purpose.

You will eventually have to get to a place in your mind where *self-care* is about making a better life that serves both you and those around you. That's the fire of love and service. It burns the longest, and it benefits everyone.

When you reach this point, tending the fire won't require near as much effort as it did in the beginning. That's when you can sit back and enjoy the heat. It's truly an amazing place to be. Most importantly, you will have a deep sense of satisfaction because you will be emotionally invested like never before.

Alignment 5: Find the Right Fit

The idea of fitness is still very personal, and in many ways misunderstood. For many people, fitness is usually one of a few things; something you do to manage your weight and body shape, something your doctor said you have to do, or an extension of your inner athlete. There are also people who exercise for mental health reasons, and some people workout so they can be "harder to kill." Yes, that's a thing.

Then there's the multidimensional maze of diet and nutrition. You can't go through a bookstore without noticing hundreds of books on dieting. Every day something will be on the morning news and talk shows about what some new study says about a certain food or vitamin. Hell, I'm a certified nutrition coach and I get tangled up in all the information myself!

Bottom line, everyone is an experiment of one, and there truly is no one-size-fits-all plan.

Your success with implementing new behaviors starts and ends with finding what works for your biology and your goals, and making it fit within your calendar and available resources.

No matter how motivated you are, or how close the gym is to your house, getting a healthy lifestyle to finally stick won't happen unless you find *what works for you*.

Along with finding what works for you, you need to acknowledge what you are willing to give up. No matter if you are trying to grow your business, grow your muscles, or grow a garden there's going to be a bill to pay. I'm not just talking about a financial bill. You will have to pay with your time and take away from other things that you may enjoy. You will have to pay with energy, mental bandwidth, and probably some degree of money, too.

Any kind of growth cycle is *resource intensive*. The bigger the goal, the bigger investment of time and resources will be required.

I don't say that to scare you off. In order to succeed, you absolutely need to have some skin in the game. Consider it functional tension. The key is knowing your risk and sacrifice tolerance in accordance with your goals. For instance, if you don't know anything about exercise or nutrition and you want to lose 100 pounds in six months, then don't expect to attain this by going to a $10-a-month gym, three times a week for an hour with no instruction.

Eventually, you will come face to face with your personal lifestyle and biology factors as well. Let me be clear, I do believe there is a special place inside each of us where we can break through so many of our limiting factors and even some of our genetic ceilings. In other words, you are much more capable of achieving big things than you think you are.

You need to be as clear as possible about your circumstances, so your goals can be adjusted if you are unable or unwilling to pay the bill. This is where most people hit the wall and quit, instead of pivoting a little bit and continuing to move forward.

Here's an example of some lifestyle factors that often need to be addressed when making your health plan fit. Let's say you are the one who usually makes the meals in the family. You want to go on a diet and lose a considerable amount of weight, but you know the rest of your family will not accept any change in your family dinner menu. Are you willing to make yourself a separate meal? Or you want to exercise but there's absolutely no time or energy left in the evening to do so? Are you willing to go to bed a little earlier so you can go to that 5:00 a.m. fitness class?

Biologically speaking, there will be factors at play that will affect how resource-intensive achieving your goals will be. Some body types are more resistant to building muscle, and some are more resistant to being thin, not to mention things like age, genetics, and other medical imbalances your body may be going through.

After reading all that, you may be like, "Geez Eric, why should I even try at all?" To which I will gladly point out that all of the obstacles above are mostly understood in the context of trying to lose weight and achieve a measurable goal. To be clear, I'm not at all opposed to losing weight or building a better-looking body, but...

I find beginners usually try to make their life fit into their goals instead of having their goals fit into their life.

I am challenging you to flip the script to see if you get the results to stick this time. After all, that's the problem this book is trying to solve. When it comes to health and fitness, we are so used to putting the cart before the horse that we don't see how the equation doesn't balance.

Being hyper-focused on the by-products of health instead of the process of integrating it, is precisely why people can't get off the yo-yo.

What if trying to make health "fit" in your life, and keep it there was your primary goal, instead of just trying to lose as much weight as possible? If you were mostly focused on *establishing consistency* at a rate your life could sustain, what kind of things would start to happen as a natural side effect? That's right, the exact things you were looking for! Once you establish consistency, then you can start to expand your capacity. That, my friends, is the magic equation.

"Consistency *before* capacity."

With behavioral change, a foundation has to be laid first. If the foundation is solid then you can build things to incredible heights. Sustainable consistency in your efforts is the foundation that all change will be built upon. In today's world, health is usually a square peg trying to fit in your "round hole" life. You need to take out the sandpaper and get to work making it slide in there.

Making small adjustments in your schedule, routine, shopping etc., can even be enjoyable, like solving a puzzle. Be patient, work small strokes and just be consistent. Change will happen faster than you realize. Just keep sanding away those edges a little bit at a time.

5.

"Food is fuel. Not the enemy, nor the therapist. Eat to live, not live to eat."

— Author Unknown

Oh food, delicious, amazing, comforting food. Food truly has a special place in our lives. Food gathering and consumption was the essence of life itself for our primitive ancestors, and we have gathered socially for meals since the dawn of time. Food even contributed to our mental health as we celebrated our kills, and felt more secure with our bellies full. Ten thousand years ago the agricultural revolution began, and growing food became the essence of power and security, as we carved off lands and borders to feed our people. This began to shape civilization as we know it today. Communities and families still revolve around food. It's both an essential element of our survival and a critical part of our social fabric.

Food consumption used to be the purpose and spoils of a hard day's work. While we still have to have jobs to pay for our food, there was something lost in translation as we stopped growing, hunting and even preparing our food.

The invention of refrigerated trucks and other extended preservation methods took the business of food to a whole new level and greatly changed our relationship with it. We created the ability to make things and keep them on the shelf longer than ever, which means less waste. That turns around and gives us a lower priced product as well. Unfortunately, as the price of mass produced, calorie dense, processed foods decrease, the cost of more natural foods like produce and meat continue to rise. All together this economic friction, coupled with increased addictive properties of processed food, and a population that was becoming more sedentary, you start to get a glimpse of some of the underlying causes of our obesity and personal health epidemics.

Personally speaking, I have tried more diets than I can count. All of them appealed to me in some way. Most of them were designed to help me cut into some next level of weight loss, or build muscle. As my thinking on nutrition matured, I became more interested in things like increasing my energy levels and keeping inflammation low, so I didn't get sick. The point I'm trying to make is nutrition, like exercise, can be adjusted to do a lot of different things to our bodies.

The problem that is plaguing many people is simply *the inappropriate relationship they have with food.*

Food is a powerful and easily accessible anesthetic for our emotions and stress.

The reward center of the brain literally lights up when sugar, fat and salt is consumed. This reward center is a deep primal mechanism in our brains that actually helped our ancestors searching for high caloric foods in order to survive.

If a caveman where to come across a piece of chocolate cake while foraging, it would be a hell of a find calorically speaking. Then he would be wired to go back to that location with some frequency hoping for more to be there. Unfortunately, chocolate cake is very easy to get a hold of now. Once again, our primal bodies are not necessarily designed to thrive in this modern world of easy access without a recalibration of our primal tendencies.

Since my first addiction was with food (it's the real gateway drug, trust me), I still struggle with its gravitational pull. I have had to come to grips with some things in order to help myself, as well as my clients, reclaim their lives and put food in its rightful place. One of the first things I had to do was start living the kind of life where I felt I was earning my food.

When I started exercising, I actually began to need food in more of a fuel capacity rather than as an anesthesia or form of entertainment.

Don't get me wrong, I'm still a sucker for a latte, but I earn them nowadays by consuming "treats" after a workout or run. Remember, the reward cycle is a part of our primal hardwiring, so why not use it to your advantage a little? We are wired to wake up, walk a long time, be patient, make the kill, and then eat. Plus, an earned reward is ten times more satisfying.

The problem with many of us is that our reward ratio is jacked up.

We simply treat ourselves way too often without earning it.

Not only does this excess do physical damage to our bodies, it does mental damage as well. Deep inside we feel like shit because we know we didn't earn that ice cream cone, or even worse, we feel terrible because we ate way more than our system needed for fuel, and now we are sluggish.

Like I mentioned before, food is an incredibly important and sophisticated part of our lives, and there are many areas to address in order for our relationship with it to evolve. Identifying the needs of nutrition, and how it interacts with your personal biology, is also a very critical step in reclaiming your health. There are foods that some people may be able to eat without issues but are toxic to their chemistry. Gas, bloating, belching, and acid reflux are not supposed to be normal body functions. They are symptoms of gastrointestinal distress, even if they came from eating "normal" food.

If you are going to get right with your health, especially in this culture, you are going to have to realize that *normal does not equal acceptable*.

Comparing what you are doing to someone else is a common mental trick we all play on ourselves. We all have said in our minds, "Well, at least I didn't order the extra-large fry like some people do." That doesn't make that medium fry you decided to order any less toxic to your system. Just because you didn't do the worst thing possible doesn't mean you moved your needle in a positive direction. Unless you always order the extra-large fry and decided to cut back, of course.

Other common "normalcy traps" are food and celebrations. Remember, just because it's a special occasion and there's food on the table doesn't mean it has to be eaten. Depending on the size of your social circle you can find yourself celebrating something quite frequently. We also need to watch out for ordering add-ons to our meal because they are offered at a lower price. Your body doesn't give a shit if getting twice as much soda for thirty more cents is a good value.

That being said, quite possibly the most destructive way "normalizing" is used is with food marketing. The food industry makes a ton of money off our general ignorance (and sometimes denial) of basic nutritional education. Never let the market educate you on anything. The market's job is to make money, not make you healthy. Often the biggest lies usually come from the "health food" section.

Words like *natural, organic, gluten free, fat free, sugar free* are all just marketing words that don't make food any more or any less healthy.

It doesn't matter if there's a farm or a sunshine on the package. What matters are the macro nutrients, ingredients, how much you consume, and whether or not your body can handle it.

Over ten years ago, my wife and I enrolled in a nutritional program with a coach. It remains one of the best things we've ever done.

She literally changed our lives and put us on a completely different trajectory for just a few hundred bucks.

The nutrition coach took us shopping and showed us how to read labels better, what to look for, and common marketing traps. She also showed us simple tips and tricks for eating better on the go, how to prepare some healthy foods we had never had before, not to mention all the other important things we didn't know about basic nutrition. Looking back, and after working with hundreds of clients, the average level of nutritional education people in our country have is what I'd consider below elementary. This is mostly due to misleading food marketing and lack of nutritional guidance from our government and even medical community. Oddly enough, doctors generally aren't trained to give nutritional advice.

Nutrition is both very simple and sophisticated. By that I mean there are a few principles that when followed will take you very far, but ultimately there is an individualized component that will always come into play. There is no single diet that works for everyone. However, here are some of those principles that will help align you with a healthier relationship with your food.

1. **Energy In vs. Energy Out**: Don't consume more than your body needs for fuel. Learn what it feels like to eat when you're hungry, as opposed to when you are bored or need stimulation. This is a HUGE step in your nutritional realignment and goes beyond counting calories, which I do not recommend. Calorie estimates for food are usually off by 20 percent or more (not in your favor), but more importantly *all calories are not equal,* meaning a 100 calories of fruit is not the same thing as a 100 calories of cake.

2. **Eat Food Not Fake Food**: There is a huge difference between real food and a "consumable product". Our bodies have a hell of a time dealing with processed foods on a biological level, and they wreak havoc

on the whole system. If you're unsure about what you're getting ready to eat just ask, "Are these ingredients something my great-great grandmother ate?"

3. **Get Your Macro-Nutrients Right**: Find out how much protein, fat and complex carbohydrates are right for your body type and goals. This is where bringing in some outside help can be a great investment if it's a confusing issue to you.

4. **Minimize Sugar and Sugar Substitutes**: These things have no nutritional value, and your body actually can't tell the difference between the real stuff and the replacements (despite what the package says). Use these sweet options as a treat *you earned*, or on very special occasions. Great-Great Grandma probably only had sugar on Sundays, if that much. Most importantly, the less you have, the better you will feel and look.

5. **Eat More Veggies Than Anything Else**. Vegetables are calorically light, have lots of fiber and are nutrient dense. They are also delicious when you learn how to prepare

them as such. Eating larger servings of vegetables is one of the best ways to shift your diet away from the unhealthy foods you love, while leaving the meal feeling satisfied.

6. **Drink Lots of Water**: Your body loves water. Not only does it help with metabolic functions for weight loss, but it also aids in higher performance and brain function. Which in turn will help you make better decisions during intense cravings. Water is also the best fuel for your system. There's a reason why you can go weeks without food, but only a couple days without water.

Even though these principles are sound, people often can find nutritional plateaus and frustrations as they move toward their goals. Every individual has unique chemistry, medical history and genetic predispositions that can come into play. Case in point, our head nutritional consultant at Seva has an assessment that includes over 300 questions just to address such issues. Sometimes getting even more in-depth testing can shed some light on those invisible obstacles.

In the end, the most important attributes to getting right with your diet will be *patience and persistence*.

No doubt, your diet is going to have to pivot and evolve, especially as your life and goals change. You may even have to bring in professionals to help get you through frustrating plateaus. There really is no end when it comes to you and your diet. It is a living and ever-changing partnership. The most critical factor is that you are *actively* participating with it and moving forward, as opposed to just mindlessly eating what sounds good and passively sliding backwards.

Step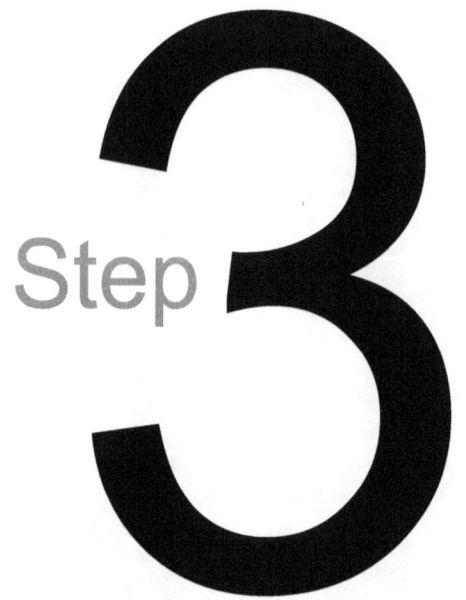

ACT

6.

"The man who moves a mountain begins by carrying away small stones."

— Confucius

The analogy of the human machine is great, but only to a point. The fact that we have a lot in common with machines provides a solid framework for an explanation of our body's maintenance requirements, but at the end of the day, we are organic beings. We operate under nature's laws, not those of technology.

Humans follow a pace of growth that mirrors that of a tree. Our rate of transformation is a comparatively slow, steady process, led by gradual changes. Obviously, cataclysmic events do occur in nature, and big shifts can speed things up. Storms can come down fast and lightning happens in a flash, but the moisture levels and elements needed for those storms to develop have to build up first. 99 percent of the time life unfolds at a very patient pace.

Something very interesting is happening to humans in the modern age. The rapid evolution of lifestyle technology - things like running water, refrigerators, microwaves, cars, phones and now the internet - have made us become intrinsically impatient when it comes to results.

When compared to the organic pace of life, our expectations are being falsely manipulated by technology. This phenomenon is stirring up unnecessarily high levels of stress, anxiety, and sometimes even delusion.

If you couple our addiction to technology with the fact that business and commerce are a huge driving force in the 21st century, the speed of life today is quite dizzying. Yet we all still must strap in and go along for the ride to some degree. While our brains are getting quite acclimated to the speed, our bodies are not. We may desire to lose weight and gain muscle rapidly,

but our nervous system and body doesn't always cooperate with our desires exactly the way we'd like them to.

As a business owner in the fitness industry, my hardest job by far is getting people to walk through my door for the first time. I answer tons of emails and phone calls from people who tell me they are gung-ho and ready to change. They want to know NOW which program might be best for them, and so on. Unfortunately, when the time comes to take the first step and actually start, something either pops up unexpectedly (subconscious sabotage, usually), or they rationalize that it's just not the right time (it's always the right time to be healthy). As much as I know their heart was in the right place, something inside of them just wasn't ready.

But my second hardest job is getting people to see the big picture, and strap in for the long haul. It may have taken them decades to get to the point they're at, yet they still have a belief that they deserve a short cut fix. How many times has this ever worked permanently?

Zero.
There are no shortcuts.

When I started taking Brazilian Jiu Jitsu, I was overly concerned with all the typical distractions, one of those being getting awarded rank in class. On my very first lesson I asked, "How long does it take to get your black belt?" When the instructor replied about 15 years I was devastated. However, I soon realized that was what made the designation so special. You were really learning how to master something, and that doesn't happen in just a couple years, or even months.

Founder and CEO of Hootsuite, Ryan Holmes explains our irrational expectations perfectly,

"You can run a sprint or you can run a marathon, but you can't sprint a marathon."

Once we get locked in on playing the long game, we become aligned with the power that small things over time really add up. Picture an archer locked in on a target a hundred yards away. What would happen if she moved her arrow just a quarter of an inch? It would go somewhere completely different. This simple lesson in trajectory is one of the most empowering truths for people who get overwhelmed trying to make changes in their lives.

If your fear of failure or inadequacy is overwhelming, simply take a smaller step. If you

keep falling short of a goal, try taking a smaller step. You are still greatly changing the outcome of your trajectory in the future.

Recently I witnessed such an occasion, where it seemed like a mile was traversed in one step, so to speak. A woman who's been dealing with overwhelming anxiety decided to come to one of our fitness classes. She knew in her head that it was something she really wanted to be able to do, because she wanted to be able to work on strength and resilience.

After a light warm up, we turned the music up and got ready to start the workout. Out of the corner of my eye I could see her take a seat while everybody else got up to begin the first exercise. I walked over and could see the tears flowing as she sat on her knees, staring ahead frozen. Looking up at me, she said, "I want to do this so bad, but it's all I can do to not run out the door right now." I told her she's doing great, we wanted her to be there, and all she needed to do was just sit and breathe. I went back to her a few more times during the workout to check on her and reassure her that everything was okay. As soon as the workout was over, she left before I could talk to her.

An hour later she actually called me to apologize, saying, "I really hope I didn't cause any drama or disruption. That was not my intention." By this heartfelt gesture alone, I could tell that she is a mindful person.

I wasn't upset at all, on the contrary, I was inspired. I told her, "You don't realize just how awesome you were today, and how big a step you took." Coming from a place of embarrassment, she naturally responded, "You really don't have to say that."

At this point I wanted to make sure she knew I wasn't just trying to make her feel better. I knew exactly how hard it was for her to stay in the class. I continued by telling her that everyone was there to challenge themselves, period.

What's challenging to one person is not necessarily challenging to another.

We all have our own battles to fight. What's most important is that we actually are facing them and trying to move forward in our lives. I guarantee that no one working out in that room was putting out as much effort as she was by resisting the urge to run. Like so many people I meet, she was holding herself to a false expectation of fitness and couldn't get past what she thought she "should" be doing, based on what she was seeing everyone else do.

We have a saying at Seva Fitness, "Keep your eyes on your own mat." The person standing next to you is a completely different person with a different history, different bone structure, different biology, different goals and different needs. There is zero benefit in comparing yourself to them.

True fitness is about taking on stress in a positive way while dealing with an elevated nervous system. That threshold is different for everyone.

Challenging ourselves appropriately and breaking our patterns is the real thing many of us are lacking. In regard to that women's personal development, she sure as hell was challenging herself by just sitting there and watching the workout. Just walking in the door that day was a complete win for her in my book.

For some of you, your next step might not be joining an exercise class; maybe it's buying an online course and working out from home for a while. Maybe it's just having a consultation with a coach. Maybe you shouldn't even start with exercise. What's most important is doing anything that would break up your routine and changing your current trajectory. After all, that's where the heart of the problem truly lies. When helping my clients with behavioral changes, I often tell them, "Just do something different." Don't worry about whether it's the right thing to do; just focus on the process of breaking up your old patterns and making better ones.

Becoming a better You is a process without an end. There are ups and downs, sure, but it is ultimately a journey without a definitive timeline, because the finish line is death, and no one knows when that is going to be.

Things like weight loss, muscle gain, running farther, lifting more weight, etc. will always be *products* of a process. You can't have a great product, or the results you want, until you've mastered the *process*.

I am a big fan of the legendary John Wooden, who many would argue is the greatest college basketball coach of all time. In a twelve-year span, as the head coach of the UCLA men's basketball team, he won ten National Championships, including seven in a row. He also holds the record for consecutive wins at eighty-eight games. But what made Coach Wooden truly legendary was his leadership style and, most importantly, his obsession with process.

Coach Wooden was once asked in a post-game interview what was going through his mind at a time when his team was behind in points. His reply was, "I was looking to see if my players were running in straight lines, or if they were running in banana patterns." He knew that if his players ran in a banana-shaped arc instead of a straight line, they would always arrive to the opportunities a tad bit slower than their opponents. This was where the rubber literally met the road (or, in this case, court) and would be one of the most defining aspects of the outcome. He never thought about the outcome first, or considered looking for shortcuts to win. It was always just about mastering the process.

Wooden had the wisdom and mental discipline to always put the cart *after* the horse.

To note the depth of Coach Wooden's process, his very first practice of the year consisted purely of teaching his players how to tie their shoes properly. From this very first lesson he built national champions.

Being process-minded isn't a groundbreaking new insight, but when it comes to building better habits it's the biggest hurdle that people lose focus on quickly, because they become target fixated. You have to learn to retrain your brain to appreciate the long game, which is all about stringing together smaller steps. And if, for some reason, you can't move forward yet, then at minimum, you can start

your process by committing to not going
backwards anymore.

As the saying goes, "If you find
yourself in a hole, the first thing to
do is stop digging."

7.

"Suck out loud."

— Ancient Punk Rock Proverb

It's remarkably unnerving to be the worst person in the room. That's one of the biggest reasons people don't want to try doing new things in their life, because nobody likes to be bad at stuff. Unfortunately, the fact remains, you have to be bad at something before you can be good at it.

It's a shame how much easier it was to do new things when we were younger. When we are kids, our sense of curiosity is profoundly more dominant than our fears and anxieties. Imagine if we still had that favoritism today. Being surrounded by new stimuli literally lights our brains up. When we allow ourselves that experience, we actually enjoy new places, people and activities. Unfortunately, our brains change, and as we *age out* of our magical and creatively limitless childhoods, we strongly begin to prefer the feelings of comfort, security and predictability. On top of that, the overwhelming responsibilities of adulthood keep piling up, and being pulled in multiple directions makes us feel like adding anything new to our lives couldn't possibly be a positive thing.

As we get older our brains acclimate to our routines, and breaking away from those routines and familiar environments are naturally accompanied with some level of anxiety.

Even when we're presented with a seemingly simple or trivial opportunity, trying anything new - no matter how small - requires a

certain level of courage from our nervous system.

Fueling the anxiety of being in a new experience is usually a feeling of embarrassment. It's important to understand that the fear of embarrassment is not just an irrational response to our feeling of adequacy; it has a much deeper origin.

Going back to a more primitive, tribal time, humans typically wouldn't want to stand out, because it might expose weakness. Doing something embarrassing could permanently cement you with a lower status in your tribe, or, even worse, cause you to be banished, which had even more serious implications. Not to mention, anything that made you stand out also made you a target. You don't have to watch many nature shows to understand that the lion is always going to go after the lone gazelle on the outskirts of the herd. Fortunately, we don't have to maintain this serious survival mentality anymore, but internal resistance to the risk that embarrassment causes can still be a very daunting obstacle.

One of Coach Scott Sonnon's most memorable lessons to me was,

"Courage always comes before confidence."

He describes confidence as a *natural by-product of repetition*, because anything we do repeatedly, we typically become better at. However, the very first act of repetition you ever undertake is usually the hardest one. It will naturally come with a sense of resistance, fear of the unknown, and a possible sense of inadequacy. Therefore, the first repetition will require a degree of courage.

Personally, I've always admired people with a natural or developed sense of adventure. To me they seem to lead the most enriching lives, and are very mentally well-adapted. My wife is one of these people. She will always chose doing something new over something routine. For myself, I don't always try new things with a sense of ease. Sometimes, I have to think about these new changes for a while, and work up the nerve to step into the unknown. Deep down, I understand that my apprehension may be completely irrational, but I allow myself some time to warm my nervous system up to the idea of the new experience. Once I've come to the conclusion that this new situation is definitely good for me, I usually go after it like jumping in cold water or tearing the band aid off.

I'm not a big fan of heights, yet I find my family constantly booking things like zipline adventures when we go on vacation. I don't find them enjoyable at all, but I use the experience to practice conquering irrational fears and managing the build-up of anxiety. I know the chances of equipment failure are ridiculously lower than getting into a car accident on the drive there, but my nervous system doesn't care.

What's critically important is that we realize *irrational resistance* to new experiences can greatly inhibit our quality of life, and even negatively impact our mental health. Then we work on it.

As anxiety rises, so does the desire for isolation, and isolating behaviors are a huge cultural obstacle right now. Technology has made it easier than ever to not have to even leave our house. More than any generation before us, we are slowly removing ourselves from our social nature, and with that comes a conditioned resistance to new experiences.

Science is strongly backing up the importance of trying new things as a foundation for brain health. *Neurobic* (neurological aerobics) exercises were created to keep the brain cognitively healthy and combat neurological deterioration. The concept is based on the idea that injecting new stimulation into our lives, no matter how seemingly simple, can have a big effect. For example, waking up to a new smell in the morning or driving a different route home from work both stimulate dormant parts of the brain, and help keep it active. As we age, this becomes even more important because our habits and routines become neurologically difficult to deviate from.

Ironically, maintaining a sense of "normalcy" makes us feel secure, but it eventually makes us less adaptable, which is the core element of survival.

Think of it this way: repeated behaviors create deeper grooves in the brain, like a wheelbarrow that has traveled the same path many times. After a while, the groove gets so deep that it's impossible to pull the wheelbarrow out and go somewhere different. This is when sayings like, "Older people get stuck in their ways", or "You can't teach an old dog new tricks" become scientifically valid. One of the biggest keys to brain health and happiness is simply *don't get stuck*.

When I took the leap and walked into a martial arts school for the first time, something in me knew that it was going to turn into something big. My brain was going in a thousand directions, and I knew this was going to be something more than simply getting in shape. Unfortunately, I was quite uncomfortable for some time. I was, without a doubt, the least capable person in the room, and after every class I had a lengthy debate with myself about quitting. Looking back, I'm quite surprised that I didn't find a reason to do it. That would've been my typical pattern. I was sore all the time; literally bruised and battered. The worst part by far was that I constantly felt like an idiot. It seemed like I was trying way too hard to get so little accomplished, but I wanted the prize that was promised with a consistent effort: becoming a better version of who I was.

Those first five years (and many instances since) were punishing to my ego and sense of security. Even though I sucked at it, I knew the training was something I absolutely needed. I felt like I was coming alive again - and truly growing - for the first time since I could remember.

I just had to make it through that initial phase and push through the suck.

We usually underestimate just how powerful new beginnings can turn out to be over time. Even something like going to a new class one hour a week can bear amazing amounts of fruit over time. Planting seeds in the ground is an activity that comes without fanfare.

As a beginner in martial arts, you are given a white belt. The color white is a symbol of your lack of experience, but it is also a symbol of purity. Your mind is likened to an empty glass, ready to be filled. As you gain wisdom and competency through the years, your belt will darken, and the black belt is the color that represents that some distinct level of competency or mastery has been achieved.

Most people think that developing attributes like toughness, precision and power are the defining qualities of the black belt, and in a way they are correct. Respected black belts are tough, and inspirational athletes. But most importantly, black belts are resilient and patient.

Resilience and patience start being established on day one, when someone allows themselves to be vulnerable enough to wear the white belt in the first place.

You could even say… "No vulnerability. No black belt."

In order to be a figurative black belt in anything functional, *vulnerability* will be a very important concept to embrace. However, it's not in our hardwiring to naturally go down that path. To our primal nervous system, allowing ourselves to be vulnerable in any way is a big no-no, and we are wired to avoid it because first and foremost we are programmed to survive.

The stoics say, "The obstacle is the way," because they understand overcoming our inherent nature is usually the key to moving from surviving to thriving.

Every great thing in our lives is born from a large degree of discomfort and humility. Until we meet this fact head-on, we are doomed to repeat our cycles and behavior patterns that are dominated by our need to be comfortable. Even when it comes to personal relationships, allowing yourself to be functionally vulnerable with people deepens the connection with them.

Consider your oldest and dearest friend: I bet they're the one who's seen you at your weakest and lowest points. In romantic relationships, the depth of vulnerability that two people allow will have a direct correlation to the level of intimacy in the partnership. Just look at the act of sex itself. What can be more vulnerable than being stripped to your bare skin, to engage in a relatively unspoken exchange where boundaries are often undefined, all while trying to figure out how to give and receive pleasure?

Sex is nerve-wracking as hell when you look at it on paper, but when inhibitions are lowered, and vulnerability is allowed, the sex is always best.

Showing up to that first fitness class, support group, book club, or whatever new endeavor that's been in the back of your mind, is going to be an instant portal into one of the most powerful pharmacies on the planet. Instant empathy and support. Deep down everyone else in the room will know how brave you were just to show up.

It's an instant steroid shot of hope. You just have to walk in the door and not close yourself off to the process.

The truth is, most fitness facilities are filled with people who, just like you, want to be better than they used to be. Every person you come across also went through that awkward first day, or struggled through that tough first year or two or three or four.

Be relentless and look for your new tribe like an excited new bride would look for a wedding dress. Try lots of things and make it exciting. Making decisions based on convenience and price alone is usually just a continuation of the same failure cycles of the past.

Having a social structure that is both supportive and challenging is critical to your success. Go somewhere where you can be challenged appropriately and grow. If it's a familiar vibe with a different coat of paint, and you feel too comfortable right away, then maybe keep looking. There are even great online communities that can get you started. Although I recommend human connection in the long run, getting started at home can be a great first step.

Many of you may be ready to jump right in. If that's where you feel you're at, then go for it. Put down this book and go sign up for something and pay online so you're committed. Make a Facebook post and tell the world you're starting that new yoga class. *Outsmart yourself* into a commitment, and back yourself into a corner you can't get out of. Embrace the feelings of anxiety and unease, because you know what they are the seeds of.

Being courageous requires fear to be present, otherwise the act wouldn't be courageous at all.

Soon you will even be able to transform the energy of anxiety into the energy of excitement. They're virtually identical energy signatures. It is taking action and responsibility for yourself that flips that switch.

It's time to cut the cord from what the old you wants to do. Remember, if you're reading this book you probably suck at this getting healthy stuff, and your instincts are shit (sorry-not sorry). Swallow that pill, because that is what productive discomfort tastes like. This is what growth looks like. You are on your way.

The first time is the worst time. Get past that and the real hard part is over. That's the obstacle. That is the way. You don't have to like it; you just have to embrace it.

When you show up on day one, *own* your rookie status. Be a proud beginner, and don't pretend to be anything else. Hell, enjoy this time. Making mistakes is expected, and you don't have to prove anything to anyone. Drop the idea that you should be good when you walk in the door. It's completely irrational; no one is holding you to that standard anyway.

Forget the speed.

Forget the destination.

Plant a seed.

Put on the white belt.

Own your rookie status.

Suck out loud.

8.

"Don't focus on what you think you deserve. Take aim on what you're willing to earn."

— David Goggins

One of the taglines we have at Seva Fitness is "Heal, Empower, Grow." The idea behind it is to show my clients that there are three phases each person cycles through in order to get right with their health. Typically, the "Heal" phase always has to come first. How quickly a person cycles through this phase depends on their starting point.

On a physical level, people need to first address negative adaptations from sitting disease and their sedentary lifestyle before they can start more moderate to intense levels of exercise. Otherwise, they will get hurt or deplete their already imbalanced system which will surely derail their progress. In the Heal phase, we have to soften and mobilize the tissue so our bones can align themselves back into a safe and strong structure. The exercises may seem less vigorous but…

Sometimes you need to take a step back to take a thousand steps forward.

On a mental level, the Heal phase consists of softening the ego in order to get an honest assessment and starting point for our journey. So many people bring to their first workouts who they used to be, or some version of who they think they should be.

In the end, most of the mental work in the Heal phase consists of people finally coming to terms with the fact that they are actually worthy of self-care, health and happiness.

This alone is a critical step for people to start moving past less important daily distractions and build a foundation that can finally move them from a surviving to a thriving mindset.

In the second phase, resilience has to be cultivated physically with discomfort in order to lay a foundation where happiness has the potential to exist. Life knocks us all down, but resilient people bounce back quicker.

Adding functional discomfort is the key element to the "Empower" phase of our model at Seva. Functional discomfort is still technically "safe," but it's not warm and fuzzy. Once we've softened and begun to heal the mind and body into a safe structure and mindset, it's then time to armor that new-found alignment.

There needs to be a hardening after the softening, because callouses ultimately help us power through in a hostile world.

Since we are creatures of comfort and survival seekers, we typically resist strenuous things on a subconscious level. The exercises and effort levels needed to make the body and nervous system adapt positively can sometimes be a little off putting for people. Activities like yoga and walking are very popular activity, but for many people I wouldn't technically consider it exercise. Don't get me wrong, they are great ways to be active and get a good mood boost, but biologically speaking, it might not technically be checking off the exercise box. Before you send me a hateful email, let me clarify my point. In the beginning, things like yoga and walking definitely can be a form of exercise, but once the body adapts results will plateau.

The magical benefits of exercise happen when our heart rates

increase and our muscles strain
to a certain threshold.

We are wired to naturally stop shy of the level of discomfort that produces transformation. This means that many people often miss out on the big medicinal dosage that fitness can provide. That's when things may need to be taken up to the next incremental notch. Working with a professional is a great way to make sure you don't get too comfortable with what is supposed to make you uncomfortable. Finding new ways to challenge yourself is absolutely essential, but it doesn't mean you have to keep adding more speed or heavier weights. Sometimes just adding new movement patterns can have a tremendous training effect, not to mention increasing sophistication in your movement is critical for brain health and fighting mental decline.

The Empower phase is about getting past doing the bare minimum, and incrementally getting your nervous system to be able to handle more stress in a healthy way. In this phase people begin to feel like they are changing on a deeper level than ever before, by simply becoming more resilient to stress. They start to see the challenge of exercise as a vehicle that's getting them where they want to go in life and helping them become the person they knew they could be.

Having more energy, focus, confidence and passion become the real fruits of your efforts. Weight loss and physique changes are just an added bonus.

The third phase is the "Grow" phase and is characterized by a strong belief and desire to be action-oriented in everything you do. Here is where you start to truly believe that the sky really is the limit.

This time it's not just a naïve flight of optimism, because you know what it takes to earn your

goals and you wouldn't have it any other way.

The biological energy system you've created gives you passionate focus from sunrise to sunset, and every small action in your day feels purposeful. You are confident you can learn whatever you need to in order to create the life you deeply desire. You still understand bad things can happen and take you off course, but that's why you train and work so hard.

You are simultaneously preparing for the hard climbs, the mudslides and the higher altitude, all while feeling a genuine sense of gratitude for your life, your health, and your mindset.

Unforeseen challenges now feel more like opportunities, and you catch your mind before it goes into negative tailspins more quickly now. Motivation comes a lot easier, and you are less distracted. It's even easier to cut some of the dead weight in your life, like acquaintances and obligations that are no longer serving you. You still have low points, but you recognize them when they are happening, not as a victim, but as a part of the human experience. This allows you to then process emotions more rapidly than ever before.

Finally, staying on track with diet and exercise is not only easier but it feels like it's as essential as oxygen. You've made the "final surrender," that the only finish line is death, and for the rest of your life you'll be an active participant.

There will be no retirement from self-betterment because in your mind you're either growing or dying.

These phases tie seamlessly together as it's hard to tell when one ends and the other begins. Also, we often have to go back through the cycle many times, like a spiral staircase going ever upward.

We live in a world that sometimes elevates short cuts by mistaking them as innovation or efficiency, but in this case, we have to let the process run its course. In the end, our happiness has to be earned as much as received. Doing the B.F.M. (Bare. Fucking. Minimum) in regard to your health will also give the Bare Fucking Minimum returns in regard to your happiness. Living passively will always catch up with you because there is no neutral on a moving train. *Life itself* is the big moving train.

It's time to get back in the game.

Take it personal.

Show up.

Fall down, get up.

Repeat until you die.

You have nothing better to do.

The finish line is death.

You are a biological machine.

Your health affects everything.

Live better.

Die slower.

Thank you very much for taking the time to read this book. This was a very special project to me, and my intention was to create something that *ignited* people into action. I want you to be healthy so you can keep focused on what's most important in your life. After all, healthy and happy people are the ones who make the world a better place.

If you would like more information for your health and fitness journey, interested in corporate wellness partnerships, or booking speaking engagements:

Please visit us at **www.LiveBetterDieSlower.com**

Connect with us on Facebook at
facebook.com/livebetterdieslower/

Or contact us at **sevamanager@gmail.com**